Fasting

By

Dr. Steve J. Hayes

Tables Of Contents

Introduction

fasting, the practice of not eating, typically for moral or religious reasons. It was employed in ancient faiths to get followers or priests ready to approach deities, to pursue a vision, to atone for misdeeds, or to calm an enraged deity. Fasting is a component of all the main global religions' traditions.

Chapter 1

Intermittent fasting

Irregular fasting is an eating plan that switches between fasting and eating on a normal timetable. Research shows that discontinuous fasting is a method for dealing with your weight and forestalling or even the opposite a few types of sickness. Yet, how would you make it happen? Furthermore, is it safe?

What is irregular fasting?

Many weight control plans center around what to eat, however, discontinuous fasting is about when you eat.

With irregular fasting, you just eat during a particular time. Research shows fasting for a specific number of hours every day or eating only once several days or seven days might have medical advantages.

Johns Hopkins neuroscientist Imprint Mattson has read up on irregular fasting for a long time. He says our bodies have advanced to have the option to do without nourishment for a long time, or even a few days or longer. In ancient times, before people figured out how to cultivate, they were trackers and finders who advanced to make due and flourish for significant stretches without eating. They needed to: It required a ton of significant investment to chase the game and accumulate nuts and berries.

Specialists note that even a long time back, keeping a solid load in the US was simpler. There were no PCs, and Network programs switched off at 11 p.m.; individuals quit eating since they headed to sleep. Segments were a lot more modest. More individuals worked and played outside and, by and large, got more activity.

With the web, television, and other amusement accessible every minute of every day, numerous grown-ups and kids stay conscious for longer hours to stare at the television, look at virtual entertainment, mess around, and talk on the web. That can mean sitting and nibbling the entire day and the vast majority of the evening.

Additional calories and less movement can mean a higher gamble of weight, type 2 diabetes, coronary illness, and different sicknesses. Logical examinations are showing that irregular fasting might assist with turning around these patterns.

How does discontinuous fasting function?

There are a few unique ways of doing discontinuous fasting, yet they are completely founded on picking customary time spans to eat and quickly. For example, you could have a go at eating just during an eight-hour time frame every day and quick for the rest of. Or on the other hand, you could decide to eat just a single dinner daily two days per week. There is a wide range of discontinuous fasting plans.

Mattson expresses that late at night without food, the body debilitates its sugar stores and starts consuming fat. He alludes to this as metabolic exchanging.

"Irregular fasting stands out from the ordinary eating design for most Americans, who eat all through their waking hours," Mattson says. "In the event that somebody is eating three dinners per day, in addition to bites, and they're not working out, then, at that point, each time they eat, they're running on those calories and not consuming their fat stores."

Irregular fasting works by delaying the period when your body has consumed the calories consumed during your last feast and starts consuming fat.

Discontinuous Fasting Plans

It means a lot to check with your primary care physician prior to beginning discontinuous fasting. When you receive their approval, genuine practice is basic. You can pick an everyday methodology, which confines day-to-day eating to one six-to eight-hour time span every day. For example, you might decide to attempt 16/8 fasting: eating for eight hours and fasting for 16.

Albeit certain individuals find it simple to stay with this example over the long haul, one exploration concentrated on that was not planned explicitly to take a gander at a discontinuous fasting design found that restricting your everyday time window of eating doesn't forestall weight gain after some time or yield huge weight reduction results. That study's outcomes showed that lessening the number of huge dinners or eating all the more little feasts might be related to limiting weight gain or even weight reduction after some time.

One more discontinuous fasting plan, known as the 5:2 methodology, includes eating consistently five days every week. For the other two days, you restrict yourself to one 500-600 calorie feast. A model would be assuming you decided to eat typically on each day of the week aside from Mondays and Thursdays, which would be your one-feast days.

Longer periods without food, like 24-, 36-, 48-and 72-hour fasting periods, are not really better for you and might be hazardous. Going excessively lengthy without eating could really urge your body to begin putting away more fat because of starvation.

Mattson's exploration demonstrates the way that it can require two to about a month prior to the body becoming familiar with discontinuous fasting. You could feel ravenous or grumpy while you're becoming acclimated to the new daily schedule. In any case, he notices, research subjects who endure the change time frame will generally stay with the arrangement since they notice they feel significantly improved.

What might I at any point eat while discontinuous fasting?

During the times when you're not eating, water and zero-calorie refreshments, for example, dark espresso and tea are allowed.

During your eating periods, "eating ordinarily" doesn't mean going off the deep end. Research shows that you're not liable to get in shape or get better assuming you pack you're taking care of times with fatty unhealthy food, super-sized broiled things, and treats.

Yet, a few specialists like discontinuous fasting that it considers a scope of various food varieties to be eaten and delighted in. Sharing great, nutritious food with others and relishing the supper time experience adds fulfillment and supports great well-being.

Most nourishment specialists view the Mediterranean eating routine as a decent outline of what to eat, regardless of whether you're attempting irregular fasting. You can scarcely turn out badly when you pick mixed greens, sound fats, lean protein, and mind-boggling, crude carbs like entire grains.

Discontinuous Fasting Advantages

Research shows that discontinuous fasting periods accomplish more than copy fat. Mattson makes sense of, "When changes happen with this metabolic switch, it influences the body and mind."

One of Mattson's examinations distributed in the New Britain Diary of Medication uncovered information about a scope of medical advantages related to the training. These incorporate a more drawn-out life, a less fatty body, and a more honed mind.

"Numerous things occur during irregular fasting that can safeguard organs against persistent sicknesses like sort 2 diabetes, coronary illness, age-related neurodegenerative issues, even incendiary entrail infection, and numerous malignant growths," he says.

Here is some discontinuous fasting benefits research has uncovered up to this point:

• Thinking and memory. Concentrates on found that irregular fasting helps working memory in creatures and verbal memory in grown-up people.

• Heart well-being. Irregular fasting further developed pulse and resting pulses as well as other heart-related estimations.

• Actual execution. Young fellows who abstained for 16 hours showed fat misfortune while keeping up with bulk. Mice who benefited from substitute days showed better perseverance in running.

• Type 2 diabetes and weight. In creature studies, irregular fasting forestalled stoutness. Also, in six brief examinations, corpulent grown-up people shed pounds by sporadic fasting. Individuals with type 2 diabetes might benefit: The majority of the accessible exploration demonstrates the way that irregular fasting can assist individuals with losing body weight and lower their degrees of fasting glucose, fasting insulin, and leptin while lessening insulin opposition, diminishing degrees of leptin and expanding levels of adiponectin. Certain examinations found that a few patients rehearsing irregular fasting with oversight by their primary care physicians had the option to switch their requirement for insulin treatment.

• Tissue well-being. In creatures, irregular fasting diminished tissue harm in a medical procedure and further developed results.

Is discontinuous fasting safe?

Certain individuals take a stab at intermitting fasting for weight executives, and others utilize the strategy to address persistent circumstances like peevish entrail condition, elevated cholesterol, or joint pain. Yet, discontinuous fasting isn't the best thing in the world for everybody.

Williams focuses on that before you attempt discontinuous fasting (or any eating regimen), you ought to check in with your essential consideration expert first.

Certain individuals ought to avoid attempting irregular fasting:

• Youngsters and adolescents under age 18.

• Ladies who are pregnant or breastfeeding.

• who use insulin and have type 1 diabetes. While a rising number of clinical preliminaries have shown that discontinuous fasting is protected in individuals with type 2 diabetes, there have been no examinations in individuals with type I diabetes. Mattson makes sense of this, "On the grounds that those with type I diabetes take insulin, there is a worry that a discontinuous fasting eating example might bring about hazardous degrees of hypoglycemia during the fasting time frame."

• Those with a background marked by dietary issues.

However, Williams says, individuals not in these classifications who can do discontinuous fasting securely can proceed with the routine endlessly. "It tends to be a way of life change," she says, "and one with benefits."

Remember that discontinuous fasting might contrastingly affect various individuals. Converse with your primary care physician in the event that you begin encountering uncommon tension, migraines, sickness, or different side effects after you start irregular fasting.

Chapter 2

Shawwal fasting

What is Shawwal?

The long stretch of Shawwal is the month following the sacred month of Ramadan and in it, there is the chance for extraordinary prizes for admirers as framed by the Courier of Allah (pbuh). Muslims have the chance to quick the six days of Shawwal, which are willful diets that can be finished whenever over time, before the finish of Shawwal. The six days of Shawwal are suggested for reclaiming any deficiencies in the nature of our diets in the long stretch of Ramadan and are identical to a time of fasting whenever acknowledged by Allah (SWT).

The principal day of Shawwal is additionally when Muslims observe Eid Al-Fitr, joining to partake in the prize of noticing the sacred month of Ramadan. This is one of the two yearly celebrations perceived by the Shari'ah. It praises the fruition of the long stretch of love:

Ramadan. Muslims go to the Eid petition on this day and pay Sadaqat ul-Fitr. It is a day of festivity.

Shawwal is the first of 90 days (before the period of Dhul Hijjah) in which a portion of the demonstrations of Hajj can start to be performed, like the Tawaf of Appearance. The time of Hajj additionally starts in Shawwal, which is generally called Debris hur Al-Hajj or the long periods of Hajj.

What purpose does Shawwal serve?

Researchers have considered a sign that a Muslim's perception of Ramadan has been acknowledged, is that they plan to quick the six days of Shawwal. As a matter of fact, Ibn Rajab (ra) said that doing so would be an approach to exhibiting our appreciation to Allah (SWT) for the endowments, leniency, and prize that Ramadan brings to the table.

"[Allah wants] for you to finish the period and to commend Allah for that [to] which He has directed you, and maybe you will be thankful" [Qur'an 2:185]

This month can likewise be a vital time for pondering the positive routines developed all through the period of Ramadan, and centering the whole self until the end of the year and then some.

Shawwal (Six Days of Shawwal) fasting

Fasting on the main day of Shawwal is restricted, in light of the fact that this is when Eid Al-Fitr happens. Be that as it may, it is prescribed to quick for six days of an admirer's picking, before the month's end to finish the six days of Shawwal and receive the benefits of an extended period of fasting.

What is the meaning of the Shawwal moon?

The locating of the new moon, or the Shawwal bow moon as it is generally called, implies the finish of the heavenly month of Ramadan, and the start of Eid al-Fitr and its celebrations. Eid al-Fitr goes on for one day, but fasting on the primary day of Eid is just restricted.

"The Prophet (harmony and favors of Allah arrive) precluded fasting upon the arrival of al-Fitr and al-Nahr."

Chapter 3

Dopamine fasting

Dopamine fasting is a type of computerized detox, including briefly going without habit-forming innovations like virtual entertainment, paying attention to music on mechanical stages, and Web gaming, and can be reached through the transitory hardship of social collaboration and eating. The term's starting points are obscure; it was first generally advanced by the holistic mentor "Improvement Pill" in November 2018 on YouTube.

The training has been alluded to as a "maladaptive craze" by one Harvard researcher. Different pundits say that it depends on a misconception of how the synapse dopamine, which works inside the cerebrum to compensate for the conduct, really works and can be modified by cognizant behavior.

The thought behind it is to have some time off from the monotonous examples of fervor and feeling that can be set off by association with computerized technology, and that the act of keeping away from pleasurable exercises can attempt to fix persistent vices, permit time for self-reflection, and support individual happiness.

Definitions

The act of dopamine fasting isn't obviously characterized by what it involves, what advances, with what recurrence it ought to be finished, or the way things should work. A few defenders limit the cycle to keeping away from online innovation; others extend it to swearing off all work, workouts, actual contact, and superfluous conversation.

As per Cameron Sepah, a defender of the training, the design isn't to in a real sense diminish dopamine in the body yet rather decrease imprudent ways of behaving that are compensated by it. One record proposes that the training is tied in with staying away from signals, for example, hearing the ring of a cell phone, that can set off hasty ways of behaving, for example, staying on the cell phone after the call to play a game. In one sense, dopamine fasting is a response to innovation firms that have designed their administrations to keep individuals hooked.

Dopamine fasting has been said to look like the fasting custom of numerous religions. An outrageous type of dopamine fasting would be finishing tangible hardship, where all outside boosts are eliminated to advance a feeling of quiet and well-being.

Effects

Defenders of dopamine fasting contend that it is a method for applying more prominent discretion and self-restraint over one's life, and New York Times innovation columnist Nellie Bowles found that dopamine fasting made her subject's day-to-day existence "seriously interesting and fun".

It has been depicted as a trend and a frenzy related to Silicon Valley. A record in Bad Habit, saying "If swearing off anything fun to build your psychological lucidity is engaging, congrats: You and the famous biohackers in Silicon Valley are on the equivalent wave."

Logical basis

Naysayers say that the general idea of dopamine fasting is informal since the substance assumes a crucial part in regular day-to-day existence; in a real sense decreasing it wouldn't be great for a person, and eliminating a specific upgrade like virtual entertainment wouldn't diminish the degrees of dopamine in the body, just the feeling of it. Ciara McCabe, Academic partner in Neuroscience at the College of Perusing, considers that the mind could be "reset" by staying away from dopamine triggers for a brief time frame to be "nonsense".

Cameron Sepah, who has advanced the act of dopamine fasting, concurs that the name is deluding and says that its motivation isn't too in a real sense diminish dopamine in the body yet rather lessen the imprudent ways of behaving that are compensated by it.

Other than the imprudent conduct control - managed by the prefrontal cortex, it's never been convincingly demonstrated that innovation use solidifies the cerebrum to dopamine's belongings. Innovation use initiates a dopamine reaction comparable to any typical, pleasant experience about a half to 100 percent expansion. On the other hand, cocaine and methamphetamine two profoundly habit-forming drugs — cause a dopamine spike of 350% and 1200% individually. What's more, dopamine receptors themselves — the cells in the mind actuated in various ways by dopamine's delivery — answer diversely to tech use than they do to substance misuse, with no proof that they become less delicate to dopamine with continuous tech use, in the manner in which they do with substance misuse. In the last examination, accepting that staying away from "dopamine spikes" may upregulate dopamine receptors, causing an "expansion in inspiration or pleasure". Alternately, liberating oneself from unfortunate behavior patterns might save time for better propensities, as actual work, prompting genuine expansions in dark matter volume on numerous cerebrum parts connected with the award system is wrong."

Chapter 4

Adjunctive fasting

Numerous patients with disease look for and utilize option and correlative therapies, meaning to work on the viability of their anticancer therapy and a decrease in therapy-related secondary effects. Momentary fasting (STF) and fasting mirroring slims down (FMDs) are among the most usually utilized dietary intercessions. Lately, various preliminaries have announced the promising aftereffects of dietary mediations in blend with chemotherapy, as far as dialing back cancer development and decrease in chemotherapy-related secondary effects. In this account survey, we distinguish and depict the ongoing proof of attainability and impacts of STF and FMDs in malignant growth patients getting chemotherapy. The examinations that analyzed the impacts of STF when joined with chemotherapy propose potential advantages in regards to a decrease in secondary effects and worked on personal satisfaction. We likewise close with a rundown of very much planned investigations that are as yet enlisting patients, looking at the drawn-out impacts of STF.

Presentation

Numerous patients with disease look for and utilize options or corresponding medicines to their normal recommended therapies. Instances of these other options and correlative medicines not just incorporate natural meds and cures and homeopathy, yet in addition healthful mediations like nutrients/minerals, restorative teas, or explicit diets.2 Patients utilize option and reciprocal medicines both with the mean to work on the viability of treatment (by supporting their resistant framework) and to decrease treatment-related side effects.1 Albeit many eating regimens exist, momentary fasting (STF) and fasting impersonating consumes fewer calories (FMDs) are presently among the most regularly utilized dietary mediations; lately, various preliminaries have revealed the fascinating aftereffects of dietary intercessions with regards to oncology.

To help and illuminate clinicians, we give a story-writing survey on FMDs integral to standard treatment for patients with the disease according to a clinical viewpoint.

What are irregular fasting and FMDs?

Irregular fasting alludes to verbose times of practically zero calorie utilization. It includes various projects that control the planning of eating events by using STF. Various examples incorporate fasting each and every other day, complete 24-h fasting, or fasting on 1 or 2 nonconsecutive days of the week. Many fasting programs exhort no or restricted caloric admission (⬚500 kcal/day) during the fasting period5 joined with a limitless number of sans-calorie drinks (for example water or espresso). The FMDs are explicit feast plans figured out to reproduce the fasting state while giving fundamental supplements and calories. They are intended to accomplish fasting-like impacts while limiting the weight of fasting. Explicit eating regimens incorporate an assortment of plant-based food varieties intended to fulfill the taste buds. Not at all like fasting, FMDs additionally give the required micronutrients like nutrients and minerals.

What pathophysiology might be impacted by fasting and FMDs?

Albeit the specific system isn't surely known, weight control by exercise and dietary calorie limitation has been related to decreased disease risk. Malignant growth cells have an unmistakable digestion, with prevalent anaerobic utilization of glucose, which is otherwise called the Warburg effect. Subsequently, fasting might distinctively affect the defenselessness of chemotherapy between sound cells and disease cells which is called differential pressure resistance. The hypothesis behind STF and FMDs is that these dietary mediations safeguard solid cells against stressors, for example, chemotherapy while making disease cells more powerless against chemotherapy and other therapies. Sound cells can switch toward an upkeep/fix state when supplements are scant/missing, (for example, during fasting), rather than malignant growth cells wherein oncogenes forestall the enactment of such pressure resistance. Fasting causes declining plasma levels of insulin-like development factor-1 (IGF-1), insulin, and glucose, all crucial in forestalling apoptosis, advancing development, and speeding up maturing, consequently prompting cancer. Notwithstanding, these impacts are possibly initiated if fasting endures for a time of no less than 48 h.

 A sub-atomic clarification for this component is that insulin and IGF-1 sign immunosuppression through the STAT3 record factor. As fasting smothers levels of circling insulin and IGFs, fasting could (hypothetically) lead to less immunosuppression and hence safe enactment, as a positive antitumor impact. Other than immunosuppression, STAT3, and the JAK-STAT3 pathways have pleiotropic impacts both as a strong cancer advertiser and as a cancer silencer factor related to cell development, apoptosis, angiogenesis, intrusion, and metastasis.

Conceivable sub-atomic pathways have been depicted to be affected by fasting and affect malignant growth science. The impact of calorie limitation on chemotherapy harmfulness was researched in vitro in typical and disease cells.19 In ordinary cells, serum starvation actuates AMPK, which balances out p53, bringing about multiplication capture. During the multiplication, capture cells are generally safeguarded from DNA-harming chemotherapy (for example CDDP). In disease cells, serum starvation also actuates the ATM/Chk2/p53 stress reaction flagging pathway. This hyperactivation of the ATM/Chk2/p53 pathway brings about over-burdening pressure which is remembered to debilitate cell stress reaction and sharpen malignant growth cells to DNA-harming chemotherapy.

In vivo, calorie limitation in mice prompted diminished action of RAS-mitogen-enacted protein kinase (MAPK) and phosphatidylinositol-3-kinase (PI3K)- AKT pathways.20 These MAPK and the PI3K/AKT flagging pathways assume a vital part in cell endurance and multiplication with an expected job in malignant growth improvement, separation, expansion, movement, and upregulation of angiogenic cytokines.21-24 The noticed inhibitory impact on RAS-MAPK and PI3K/AKT pathways gives a potential connection between the disease counteraction by the utilization of calorie limitation. These preclinical discoveries connected with sub-atomic flagging demonstrate that calorie limitation might possibly upgrade the remedial impact of DNA-harming chemotherapy.

What is the preclinical proof for FMDs?

In preclinical examinations in mice, FMDs forestalled age-related sicknesses, exhibited improved irritation, and metabolic profile, and expanded the life expectancy of the mice.6 Besides, patterns of starvation were pretty much as viable as chemotherapeutic specialists in deferring movement of various growth models and expanded the viability of chemotherapy in melanoma, glioma, and bosom disease cells. In mouse models of neuroblastoma, fasting cycles in addition to cytotoxic medications, yet not either therapy alone, brought about long haul malignant growth-free survival. In mouse models with chemical receptor-positive bosom malignant growth treated with chemical treatment, FMD likewise makes positive impacts, prompting a dependable cancer relapse and forestalling tamoxifen-instigated endometrial hyperplasia. In another bosom disease mouse model (metastatic triple-negative bosom malignant growth of mice infused with 4T1-luc cells), patterns of FMD essentially dialed back growth development, diminished cancer size, and caused an expanded articulation of intratumoral Caspase3, recommending enactment of apoptosis. This concentrate additionally showed less dispersed metastasis with prevalent lung metastasis in FMD mice, versus more scattered, different organ and lymph hub metastasis in typical eating routine mice. Close to critical development delay, even total reductions were accounted for in a piece of the mesothelioma xenografts (60%) and lung carcinoma xenografts (40%) following fasting. Other than viability, mice models likewise showed fasting shielded from leukopenia, heart, kidney, and liver harm when abstained for 24 h previously and 24 h after oxaliplatin or doxorubicin administration. By and large, preclinical examinations have exhibited the promising impacts of fasting and FMDs on chemotherapy viability and security in regard to secondary effects.

What are the immunomodulatory impacts of fasting and FMD?

Fasting and FMDs have been exhibited to regulate the safe reaction by different instruments. One component exhibited in a murine bosom disease and melanoma model shows that FMDs improve the collection of growth penetrating lymphocytes and Lymphocyte intervention in cancer cytotoxicity. Besides, STF reduces the degrees of circling IGF-1 to sharpen growths to customized cell demise protein 1 bar in preclinical models of non-little cell lung cancer, expanding malignant growth immunogenicity, and helping antitumor CD8 Immune system microorganism responses. In low-immunogenic triple-negative bosom disease models, two patterns of a 4-day FMD were joined with either hostile to modified passing ligand 1 (PD-L1) or a mix of against OX40 (costimulatory receptor) and hostile to PD-L1. FMD changed the digestion from glycolysis to oxidative phosphorylation reshaping the cancer miniature climate and improving the viability of immunotherapy in TNBC growth types. A similar report likewise showed an FMD-prompted decrease in safe-related unfavorable occasions (AEs) by forestalling hyperactivation of the resistant reaction. This is a promising healthful mediation that could be applied to sharpen low-immunogenic cancers to immunotherapy.

What could be generally anticipated by STF and FMDs from a clinical pharmacology viewpoint?

STF and FMDs present significant pharmacokinetic communications in regard to retention and digestion. The retention is particularly applicable for oral-formed oncolytic medications, for example, capecitabine [but likewise for S1, and past chemotherapy for oral (designated) treatments, including tyrosine kinase inhibitors (TKIs)]. For oral chemotherapy, for example, the rate (Tmax) and sum [Cmax and region under the bend (AUC)] of capecitabine are a lot higher when taken in abstained conditions. The solvency of, for example, TKIs is to a great extent reliant upon the intragastric sharpness (pH Level). Food in the stomach can cradle causticity, accordingly expanding intragastric pH. This postprandial intragastric expansion in pH can diminish the dissolvability and retention of a portion of these drugs. For other, for instance, lipophilic medications, corresponding high-fat dinners can fundamentally increment plasma concentrations, exemplified by lapatinib's AUC is 425% (after ingestion with a high-fat feast contrasted with the fasting state.) These noticed contrasts in bioavailability and outright changeability warrant individual proposal in regards to food-fasting and medication collaborations in little particles for which an outline is given by Veerman et al. Even inside one medication class, contrasts exist. For instance, consolidating fasting and organization of the oral CDK4/6 inhibitor palbociclib brought about lower levels and less unsurprising pharmacokinetic fluctuation. Thusly, the suggestion is that palbociclib ought to be managed with food. For the other CDK4/6 inhibitors ribociclib and abemaciclib, the impacts of fasting on drug openness are insignificant.

Concerning digestion, fasting has been displayed to impact fundamental medication digestion by both prompting specific cytochrome P450 (CYP) and UGT proteins (CYP1A2, CYP2D6 CYP3A4, UGT1A4, and UGT2B4/2B7) and decreasing chemical action of others (2C9).38 Albeit these impacts seem, by all accounts, to be restricted (12-20%), for cytotoxic specialists with overall little restorative ranges, these fasting-initiated changes could be clinically pertinent. In one of the included examinations, restorative medication observation was accounted for; in this review, irinotecan plasma levels were estimated and displayed following protein and calorie limitations. The openness to irinotecan and its dynamic metabolite SN-38 demonstrated as AUC from zero to 24 h (AUC 0-24 h), was 7.1% and 50.3% higher after protein and calorie limitation versus an

ordinary eating regimen, without critical expansion in grade ⬚ 3 toxicity.

Are STF and FMD during chemotherapy protected and practical?

STF from 48 human individuals (n = 10-131) receiving various growth-specific chemotherapeutic regimens participated in six small studies. to 140 h before and 5-56 h following chemotherapy was all around endured, safe, and feasible, while diminishing its poisonousness.

Fasting for 48 h is very much endured without expanding weight reduction, clinic confirmations, or chemotherapy portion decrease/delays as per a randomized control preliminary in ladies with gynecologic malignancies getting no less than six arranged chemotherapy cycles.

Fasting patients keeping a water-just quick for 24 h previously and 24 h following every chemotherapy cycle were contrasted with non-fasting patients. Treatment-related incidental effects and personal satisfaction (QoL) were surveyed utilizing the NCCN-Reality FOSI-18 poll. The vast majority of the patients got taxane-and platinum-based doublet treatment. Weight reduction and unexpected hospitalizations were comparable between treatment gatherings. There were fewer portion decreases or postpones enlisted in the fasting gathering and fasting didn't bring about huge weight reduction, even in a patient populace at critical gamble for malnutrition.

A case series of 10 patients with various malignancies going through treatment joined with STF likewise exhibited the security and practicality of STF. Each of the 10 cases abstained for 48-140 h preceding and additionally 5-56 h following chemotherapy. None of these patients, who got a normal of four patterns of different chemotherapy drugs in the mix with fasting, detailed huge secondary effects brought about by the actual fasting other than hunger and lightheadedness.

In another clinical review assessing wellbeing, bearableness, and QoL of consolidating chemotherapy with STF, better resistance to chemotherapy was reported11. This study included ladies with bosom malignant growth and ovarian disease and utilized an intra-individual randomized get-over to concentrate on a plan to adjust for the heterogeneity in illness states and chemotherapy conventions. STF with a time of 60 h was not related to weight reduction and was related to just minor unfriendly impacts that were evaluated as not significant by the patients and didn't slow down everyday exercises.

When joined with chemotherapy and standard antineoplastic therapies in disease patients at low healthful gamble, occasional FMD cycles are feasible.

What is the adequacy of irregular fasting and FMDs with respect to security against poisonousness and chemotherapy-related secondary effects?

Various examinations have researched the viability of FMDs concerning security against harmfulness, chemotherapy-related secondary effects, and QoL.

 A randomized control preliminary was directed at ladies with gynecologic malignancies getting no less than six arranged chemotherapy cycles joined with STF. Fasting during chemotherapy prompted an improvement in persistent revealed QoL scores throughout chemotherapy treatments.40 Albeit this study was not controlled to recognize further contrasts in results, there was a pattern toward fewer hospitalizations, improvement in hematologic boundaries, and fewer portion decreases or postpones in treatment for the fasting bunch.

In a little and heterogeneous gathering of patients during and after Ramadan, fasting was very much endured and a practically identical decrease in secondary effects contrasted with the non-fasting period was reported. Eleven disease patients getting chemotherapy were enlisted for this pilot study. Patients were permitted to proceed with their normal fasting plan while getting chemotherapy. After a 'wash out' time of no less than about fourteen days after the finish of Ramadan, patients

got similar chemotherapy while not fasting. All patients were evaluated by telephone day to day with respect to possible chemotherapy incidental effects, and total blood consideration well as renal and liver capability were observed once week after week. All patients announced fewer secondary effects in the chemotherapy period during Ramadan.

In ladies with bosom disease and ovarian malignant growth, STF prompted a superior resilience to chemotherapy with less compromised QoL (FACIT-estimation framework) and diminished exhaustion 8 days after chemotherapy. In this randomized get-over preliminary, gynecologic disease patients with four to six arranged chemotherapy cycles were incorporated. On the whole, 34 patients were randomized to STF in the main portion of chemotherapy treatment followed by a noncaloric diet (bunch A; n = 18) or the other way around (bunch B; n = 16). Fasting began 36 h previously and finished 24 h after chemotherapy (60-h fasting period).

Close to better chemotherapy resistance, STF was not related to any serious side effects.11 Comparable discoveries were accounted for in an investigation of 13 ladies with HER2-negative bosom malignant growth who were treated with chemotherapy. Qualified patients with HER2-negative stage II/III bosom disease getting (neo)-adjuvant chemotherapy (docetaxel/doxorubicin/cyclophosphamide) were randomized to quick 24 h when starting chemotherapy, or to eat as per the rules for solid sustenance. Chemotherapy-prompted DNA harm in fringe blood mononuclear cells (PBMCs) was measured by the degree of γ-H2AX (a delicate sub-atomic marker of DNA harm and fix) broke down by stream cytometry. STF was very much endured and mean erythrocyte and thrombocyte counts following 7 days of chemotherapy were fundamentally higher in the STF bunch contrasted with the non-STF bunch. Levels of γ-H2AX were essentially expanded 30 min post-chemotherapy in CD45+ CD3− cells in non-STF, but not in STF patients. STF might lessen a transient increment or potentially prompt a quicker recuperation of DNA harm in PBMCs after chemotherapy. Non-hematologic harmfulness didn't contrast between the gatherings.

The Immediate preliminary research on the impact of the expansion of an exceptional a low-calorie and protein-limited diet (Chemolieve) to chemotherapy on incidental effects and impact of chemotherapy (four courses of AC followed by four courses of docetaxel) in patients with bosom cancer. On the whole, 131 patients with HER2-negative stage II/III bosom malignant growth were randomized to get either an FMD or their standard eating regimen for 3 days before and during neoadjuvant chemotherapy. Results showed no distinction in harmfulness between the two gatherings, in spite of the way that dexamethasone was precluded in the FMD bunch. FMD might mitigate the requirement for prophylactic treatment with dexamethasone for the avoidance of chemotherapy incidental effects. Consequences of the auxiliary results of the DIRECT trial48 detailed improvement of specific QoL and ailment discernment spaces in patients getting FMD as an assistant to neoadjuvant chemotherapy. The occurrence of extreme harmfulness (Normal Wording Models for Unfavorable Occasion grade ⍰ 3) in patients treated with irinotecan on a protein and calorie limitation appeared to be higher (53%) contrasted with a typical eating routine

(42%), albeit this pattern was not genuinely unique (p = 0.69).39

In the latest concentrate by Vernieri et al., 10 patients getting n with standard antitumor treatments were relegated to a cyclic 5-day FMD routine. The preliminary detailed great consistency and no expanded security concerns. The preliminary met its essential endpoint, with a frequency of serious grade 3 or 4 FMD-related AEs of 12.9% (90% certainty span: 7.8-19.7%), fundamentally lower than the pre-indicated 20% threshold.4 A practically identical well-being profile was seen by Valdemarin et al. In this single-arm, stage I/II clinical preliminary, 100 patients with strong or hematologic threat went through dynamic clinical treatment joined with occasional FMD cycle. No grade 3-5 AEs connected with FMD were noticed.

What is the impact of STF on the reaction to chemotherapy?

There is just a single randomized controlled concentrate that has assessed the impacts of an FMD on the viability of chemotherapy in human patients with malignant growth (DIRECT preliminary, depicted in the past section). A FMD worked on the clinical reaction to neoadjuvant chemotherapy when contrasted with a customary eating regimen in HER2-negative early bosom malignant growth patients getting chemotherapy. Radiologically complete or fractional reaction happens all the more frequently in patients utilizing the FMD [odds proportion (OR): 3.168, p = 0.039] and an obsessive reaction was bound to happen in patients utilizing the FMD (OR: 4.109, p = 0.016). The consequences of DIRECT preliminary showed the way that FMDs could make dexamethasone pre-drug pointless in anticipation of chemotherapy-actuated sickness and vomiting. This could be vital in light of the fact that glucocorticoids including dexamethasone are remembered to advance bosom malignant growth metastasis. By keeping away from dexamethasone, FMDs might hence actually fortify the anticancer impacts of chemotherapy.

What is the ideal term for FMD or STF?

The span of fasting time frames in the various examinations went from 48 to 140 h.11,12,42,44,45 This is the main review that assessed various regimens/lengths of STF during the examination of 20 patients with three different fasting periods (24, 48, and 72 h).45 In this preliminary, 16 of the patients were agreeable with the fasting routine (<200 kcal/day) and showed diminished DNA harm in (host)leukocytes after chemotherapy openness for subjects who abstained 72 h contrasted with 24 h. For the FMDs, four preliminaries assessed practically identical terms of FMDs of 4 days12 (DIRECT preliminary) and 5 days,4,43,47 The included growth types in these examinations varied. The 5-day FMD routine showed superior adherence, albeit the noticed contrast could be made sense of by the different calorie content and patient qualities varied (see Table 1 and separate subheading).

What is the ideal FMD routine?

Most investigations assessing FMDs all had a bi-phasic routine of 4-5 days with a medium limitation on Day 1 with additional caloric limitation on the next days. Dietary items in the FMDs fluctuate and go somewhere in the range of 1200 and 600 kcal on Day 1 followed by a limitation somewhere in the range of 700 and 200 kcal/day. roughly 1099 kcal on Day 1 (11% protein, 46% fat, and 43% sugars), roughly 717 kcal (9% protein, 44% fat, and 47% carbs) on Days 2-5.47 The Immediate review FMD routine contained 1200 kcal on Day 1 and 200 kcal on Days 2-4. In the latest distribution by Vernieri et al., a 5-day FMD routine including 600 kcal on Day 1, up to 300 kcal on Days 2-5 was applied. Most FMDs comprise plant-based fixings and the wholesome items differ

Consistency is a significant issue in regard to FMD use in the mix with chemotherapy. It shifted between studies. Not at all like the Immediate preliminary that revealed poor FMD consistency of 20% for all arranged FMD cycles,12 other late human oncologic and non-oncologic preliminaries have announced much better consistence of up to 72%. These noticed contrasts in consistency could be made sense of by contrasts in the FMD piece and patient administration. Given the heterogeneity and nature of the revealed preliminaries, with no holds barred examinations, the ideal FMD routine including the timing, how much caloric limitation, and which supplements ought to be confined/saved is obscure.

Which patients were remembered for STF and FMD preliminaries?

The clinical preliminaries depicted in this article will generally recommend a positive pattern on the side of the mix in patients getting disease treatment for various malignancies. When joined with chemotherapy, STF or FMD could give therapy-related benefits to intolerant patients with bosom cancer and gynecologic cancers. The two latest preliminaries were less specific as they remembered patients with >10 various malignancies for various anticancer therapy.

Which clinical preliminaries of FMDs and STF are progressing inside clinical oncology?

As the field of clinical oncology and correlative eating regimens is quickly developing, we sum up the enrolled preliminaries exploring FMDs and STF inside clinical oncology. We distinguished nine preliminaries as of now enrolled with various oncologic circumstances (lung, bosom, ovarian, prostate, and colorectal malignant growth) going from stage II to arrange IV. The essential endpoints are obsessive reaction, QoL, ideal fasting term, and grade 2-4 aftereffects. The normal number of members fluctuates per study going from 12 to 150 members with an assessed concentration on the finish date going from 2022 to 2024.

End and future headings

Out and out, STF and FMDs are promising dietary mediations; nonetheless, vulnerability continues with respect to the security, attainability, and viability of fasting in the reaction to chemotherapy for everybody.

Particularly STF including water-possibly fasting can present well-being issues when supported for a more drawn-out time frame and can decrease adherence. In light of past preliminaries, explicit information holes in writing incorporate the ideal fasting plan (timing, the measure of caloric limitation, and which supplements ought to be confined). Preferably, an enormous randomized clinical preliminary would look at the normalized FMD and a control arm a typical eating routine all joined with standard chemotherapy with movement-free endurance, in general endurance, and secondary effects as its endpoints. Such a preliminary would preferably have to incorporate an action to survey consistency. The noticed consistency in late preliminaries exhibits high FMD consistency can be reached by dietician support. Everything being equal, such preliminaries are difficult to subsidize and coordinate and individualized guiding of patients with respect to their desires for correlative consideration ought to stay the norm of care. Medical care experts in oncology ought to hence be sufficiently educated regarding the dangers and advantages of dietary mediations as reciprocal malignant growth therapy.

Chapter 5

Autophagy

Autophagy is a characteristic, self-protection component by which the body eliminates harmed or useless pieces of a cell and reuses different parts toward cell fix.

Autophagy is the body's approach to wiping out harmed cells, to recover more up-to-date, better cells, as per Priya Khorana, PhD, in sustenance schooling from Columbia College.

"Auto" signifies self and "phagy" signifies eat. So the strict importance of autophagy is "self-eating."

It's additionally alluded to as "self-gobbling up." While that might seem like something you never need to happen to your body, it's really gainful to your general well-being.

This is on the grounds that autophagy is a developmental self-protection system through which the body can eliminate the broken cells and reuse portions of them for cell fix and cleaning, as indicated by a board-confirmed cardiologist, Dr. Luiza Petre.

Petre makes sense that the reason for autophagy is to eliminate trash and self-control back to ideal smooth capability.

"It is reusing and cleaning simultaneously, very much like hitting a reset button on your body. Furthermore, it advances endurance and variation as a reaction to different stressors and poisons gathered in our cells," she adds.

What are the advantages of autophagy?

The fundamental advantages of autophagy appear to come as hostile to maturing standards. As a matter of fact, Petre says all that needs to be said is known as the body's approach to turning the clock back and making more youthful cells.

Khorana brings up that when our phones are worried, autophagy is expanded to safeguard us, which helps improve our life expectancy.

Moreover, enlisted dietitian, Scott Keatley, RD, CDN, expresses that in the midst of starvation, autophagy moves the body along by stalling cell material and reusing it for essential cycles.

"Obviously this takes energy and can't go on perpetually, yet it gives us an additional opportunity to track down sustenance," he adds.

At the cell level, Petre says the advantages of autophagy include:

• eliminating harmful proteins from the cells that are credited to neurodegenerative illnesses, like Parkinson's and Alzheimer's sickness

• reusing leftover proteins

• giving energy and building blocks to cells that may as yet profit from fix

• for a bigger scope, it prompts recovery and sound cells

Autophagy is getting a ton of consideration for the job it might play in forestalling or treating disease, as well.

"Autophagy declines as we age, so this implies cells that never again work or may cause damage are permitted to increase, which is the MO of disease cells," makes sense Keatley.

While all tumors start from some kind of deficient cells, Petre says that the body ought to perceive and eliminate those cells, frequently utilizing autophagic processes. That is the reason a few scientists are taking a gander at the likelihood that autophagy may bring down the gamble of disease.

While there's no logical proof to back this up, Petre says some studiesTrusted Source recommends that numerous harmful cells can be eliminated through autophagy.

"This is the manner by which the body polices the disease, bad guys," she makes sense of. "Perceiving and obliterating what turned out badly and setting off the fixing system adds to bringing down the gamble of disease."

Specialists accept that new investigations will prompt understanding that will assist them with focusing on autophagy as a treatment for the disease.

Diet changes that can help autophagy

Recollect that autophagy in a real sense signifies "self-eating." In this way, it's a good idea that discontinuous fasting and ketogenic counts calories are known to set off autophagy.

"Fasting is [the] best-way to set off autophagy," makes sense Petre.

"Ketosis, an eating routine high in fat and low in carbs brings similar advantages of fasting without fasting, similar to an alternate route to prompt similar valuable metabolic changes," she adds. "By not overpowering the body with an outside load, it offers the body a reprieve to zero in on its own wellbeing and fixes."

In the keto diet, you get around 75% of your everyday calories from fat, and 5 to 10 percent of your calories from carbs.

This change in calorie sources makes your body shift its metabolic pathways. It will start to involve fat for fuel rather than the glucose that is gotten from carbs.

In light of this limitation, your body will start to begin creating ketone bodies that make numerous defensive impacts. Khorana says studies propose that ketosis can likewise cause starvation-initiated autophagy, which has neuroprotective capabilities.

"Low glucose levels happen in the two weight control plans and are connected to low insulin and high glucagon levels," makes sense Petre. What's more, the glucagon level is the one that starts autophagy.

"At the point when the body is falling short on sugar through fasting or ketosis, it brings the positive pressure that awakens the endurance fixing mode," she adds.

One non-diet region that may likewise assume a part in prompting autophagy is working out. As per one creature study, actual activity might actuate autophagy in organs that are important for metabolic guideline processes.

This can incorporate the muscles, liver, pancreas, and fat tissue.

The primary concern

Autophagy will keep on acquiring consideration as specialists direct more investigations on the effect it has on our well-being.

Until further notice, dietary and wellbeing specialists, for example, Khorana highlight the way that there's still a lot of we really want to find out about autophagy and how to best support it.

Yet, in the event that you're keen on attempting to animate autophagy in your body, she suggests beginning by adding fasting and standard activity into your daily schedule.

In any case, you want to counsel your primary care physician in the event that you're taking any meds, are pregnant, breastfeeding, wish to become pregnant, or have an ongoing condition, like coronary illness or diabetes.

Khorana alerts that you're not urged too quickly assuming you fall into any of the above classifications.

What occurs during autophagy?

Autophagy-related proteins (ATGs) make autophagy conceivable. Autophagosomes are formed as a result of ATGs. Autophagosomes convey the garbage cell parts of a piece of the phone called a lysosome. A lysosome's responsibility is to process or separate other cell parts.

Envision lysosomes — part of a cell — eating different pieces of the cell. "Autophagy" is a mix of two Greek words meant to imply "self-eating up":

• "Automobiles" signifies self.

• "Phagomai" signifies to eat.

Lysosomes eat the garbage cell parts and afterward, discharge the reusable pieces and pieces. The cells utilize these unrefined substances to make new parts.

What causes autophagy?

Autophagy happens when your body's cells are denied supplements or oxygen or on the other hand assuming that they're harmed somehow or another.

Think about it along these lines: Autophagy is a reusing interaction that capitalizes on a cell's now-existing energy assets. The interaction slopes up when your body needs to take advantage of these assets in light of the fact that your cells aren't getting them from an external source.

With autophagy, a cell basically eats itself to make due. The reward is that this endurance cycle can prompt cells that work all the more proficiently.

Could you at any point initiate autophagy?

You can initiate autophagy by focusing on your cells to send them into endurance mode. You can actuate autophagy through:

• Fasting: Fasting implies that you quit eating for a specific measure of time. Fasting denies your assemblage of supplements, compelling it to reuse cell parts to work.

• Calorie limitation: Confining your calories implies diminishing the number of energy units, or calories, your body consumes. Rather than denying your collection of calories totally (similarly to fasting), you restrict them.

This powers your cells into autophagy to make up for the lost supplements.

• Changing to a high-fat, low-carb diet: This kind of diet, generally alluded to as a keto diet, fundamentally impacts the manner in which your body consumes energy so that as opposed to consuming carbs or sugar for energy, it consumes fat all things considered. This switch can set off autophagy.

• Work out: Exercise animates processes that increment the action of ATGs, for example, focusing on your skeletal muscles. Exercise can actuate autophagy, contingent upon the kind of activity you're doing and its power.

All things considered, having the option to instigate autophagy doesn't mean you ought to. For example, fasting, calorie limitation, or changing to a keto diet may not be protected in the event that you're pregnant, breastfeeding, or on the other hand in the event that you have a condition like diabetes. Essentially, you shouldn't start an incredible workout daily practice without speaking with a medical care supplier.

How much time must pass before autophagy occurs?

Animal studies suggest that autophagy may begin between 24 and 48 hours after a fast.

 Insufficient exploration has been gathered on the ideal timing to set off human autophagy.

Converse with a medical services supplier in the event that you're thinking about massive changes to your eating regimen, such as fasting. While fasting might be a decent choice for certain individuals, it might jeopardize others' well-being. Try not to take a chance with it.

What is the connection between autophagy and illness?

Researchers once considered autophagy as housekeeping — your cells' approach to cleaning up to get by and capability accurately. In the beyond 20 years, researchers have found that autophagy may likewise assume a significant part in forestalling and answering sickness.

For example, studies definitely dislike autophagy might be related with:

- Crohn's illness.

- Diabetes.

- Coronary illness.

- Huntington's illness.

- Kidney illness.

- Liver illness.

- Parkinson's illness.

Issues with autophagy are likewise connected with disease. "Garbage" gathering in a phone might expand the gamble of blunders in a phone's hereditary material or DNA. Hereditary transformations, or changes, in cell DNA, can prompt malignant growth cell shaping.

In any case, autophagy is definitely not an obvious hurtful or helpful cycle concerning illness counteraction or treatment. For example, a few examinations have shown that autophagy may keep growths from framing in the beginning phases of the disease. Another exploration has shown that autophagy may empower growth development by assisting disease cells with working all the more productively.

Likewise, most examinations about the connection between autophagy and illness haven't been performed on people. Most testing has concentrated on creatures, similar to mice or rodents, who (like all vertebrates) experience autophagy.

As researchers gather more proof about the connection between autophagy and illness, we'll find out how this cycle might assume a part in specific circumstances and long-haul wellbeing.

Chapter 6

Omad fasting

Eating one feast a day (OMAD) is an eating routine arrangement that might bring about weight reduction. While that might seem like something worth being thankful for assuming you want to get thinner, it's fundamental to consider what this kind of eating example can mean for your wellbeing. This is the thing you really want to be aware of the OMAD diet

What Is the One Dinner Daily Eating Regimen (OMAD)?

A type of fasting is the One Feast a Day diet.

 Fasting is characterized as going without eating food and calorie-containing drinks for a while.

There are two standard sorts of discontinuous fasting that slim down - time-confined taking care (TRF) and substitute-day fasting (ADF). Models incorporate fasting for 16 hours followed by an eight-hour eating period and fasting on substitute days. Discontinuous fasting slims down one normal component enjoying intermittent reprieves from eating.

With OMAD, just a single dinner is eaten for the entire day, which makes sense L.J. Amaral, an enrolled clinical and research dietitian at Cedars-Sinai in Los Angeles spends significant time in disease nourishment research and ketogenic and fasting-impersonating eats less.

How Does the OMAD Eat Less Work?

The one feast eaten on the OMAD diet is generally consumed around supper time, says Amaral.

"You quick the entire day for up to 22 to 23 hours," notes Ella Davar, an enlisted dietitian and wellbeing guide situated in New York City. In any case, non-calorie refreshments, for example, water and espresso are permitted over the course of the day, she adds.

"There are not really calorie limitations, but rather a great many people attempt to fit all of their [nutritional] needs in this one feast," makes sense Amaral.

"Discontinuous fasting has been displayed to assist people with shedding pounds," says Joan Salge Blake, EdD, a nourishment teacher at Boston College and host of the sustenance and wellbeing webcast, SpotOn! "Nonetheless, OMAD is an outrageous form. Weight reduction will probably happen as calories will be confined," she notes, making sense of squeezing all your calorie and supplement needs into one meal can be troublesome.

There are no rules on the kind of food to eat and no food limitations with the OMAD diet. All things considered, Dr. Salge Blake says "The dinner can contain any food, which can make it undesirable." For instance, she adds that an individual "could devour treats and cakes" in one feast, making it a sugar-rich dinner.

Advantages of Fasting

Concentrates on well-defined one feast a day or diminished dinner recurrence are restricted. In any case, discontinuous fasting overall has been displayed to offer potential medical advantages.

Weight reduction

"Fasting is a powerful method for assisting you with losing fat," notes Davar. For sure, time-confined eating (TRE) was noted to prompt a deficiency of fat mass, as well as a 3% normal weight reduction, in a 2020 Supplements study looking at 23 clinical preliminaries on the well-being impacts of TRE (where the eating time frame is limited to 10 hours or less with a fasting time of 14 hours or more)[1]. Strangely, the fat misfortune was seen with next to no limitation on calorie consumption.

Well defined for diminished feast recurrence, a 2017 Diary of Nourishment study with more than 50,000 members reasoned that a short-term quick of 18 to 19 hours with a five to six-hour eating window that included two dinners, preferably breakfast, and lunch, might be a useful procedure for weight control.

Advantageous Metabolic Impacts

In the previously mentioned Supplements survey, the accompanying gainful metabolic impacts were seen with TRE, outstandingly with a fasting time of 16 hours. Scientists likewise saw that these impacts might be created freely of calorie consumption. The examination proposes that nourishment influences well-being through diet quality and amount as well as through the planning of dinners.

• Diminished glucose level

• Further developed insulin obstruction

• Lower fatty oil level

• Expansion in HDL (great) cholesterol

• Diminished systolic pulse

Against Disease Procedure

Fasting may likewise assist with disease treatment, notes Amaral. Be that as it may, while research in this space is promising, it's still at its outset. In a 2020 Worldwide Diary of Sub-atomic Sciences survey, scientists make sense of that fasting when chemotherapy can assist with the viability and decency of chemotherapy by empowering the endurance of typical cells while destroying malignant growth cells. The creators presumed that huge randomized control preliminaries are expected to lay out well-being and efficacy.

Dangers of OMAD Diet

While specialists concur that there are advantages to irregular fasting, they additionally note the dangers of the OMAD diet and fasting overall.

The OMAD diet's serious limitation "may prompt confused eating and make it incredibly testing to meet everyday supplement needs for nutrients, minerals, and fiber," alerts Dr. Salge Blake.

"Fasting for over 14 hours might make certain individuals experience a higher pressure reaction, crabbiness, and lower glucose," notes Davar.

"Low glucose can incorporate side effects, for example, unsteadiness, migraines, precariousness, raised pulse and narrow-mindedness to cold," makes sense of Amaral who proceeds to say that the OMAD diet could likewise prompt lack of hydration.

Extra dangers include:

• Quicker weight reduction than is considered protected by specialists

• Insufficient calories (under 1,200 calories)

• OMAD diet doesn't show good dieting propensities

• The eating routine is challenging to maintain, especially in friendly circumstances

• One dinner daily is contraindicated in individuals with diabetes or who are on sure prescriptions that should be taken with food during the day

Who Could Profit From Attempting the OMAD to Eat fewer carbs?

Irregular fasting overall can be valuable for individuals who are living with metabolic conditions, those with marginal diabetes, as well as individuals attempting to get in shape, says Amaral.

Intended for the OMAD diet, Davar takes note of that "it could be gainful to integrate for one to two days per week, to check whether it's something that your body answers well to." It might likewise be useful for occupied individuals with requesting hours or somebody who's as of now experienced irregular fasting and sees the advantages, she notes. In any case, she suggests beginning with less prohibitive types of irregular fasting like fasting for 14 to 16 hours with a few feasts. Continuously make certain to talk with an enrolled dietitian or clinical expert prior to beginning such an eating routine.

Who Ought to Try not to Attempt the OMAD to Consume fewer calories?

While Dr. Salge Blake concurs with the general advantages of less prohibitive discontinuous fasting, she doesn't prescribe the OMAD diet explicitly to anybody. "There are alternate ways of improving [health markers] and getting thinner without such a serious limitation," she expresses, proceeding to take note that she inclines toward feast timing. "Eating a greater amount of your calories in the day and tightening them as the day goes on can influence your weight and other [health] markers," Dr. Salge Blake keeps, referring to a 2013 Corpulence Society randomized study[4]. The advantages of dinner timing are likewise outlined in a fresher 2021 Supplements review.

Dr. Salge Blake exhorts against discontinuous fasting slims down for the accompanying gatherings.

• Developing people like youngsters and teenagers

• Individuals who are pregnant or breastfeeding

• More seasoned grown-ups

• Individuals with a background marked by scattered eating

• Individuals with diabetes

Since fasting can possibly influence glucose and circulatory strain, Amaral doesn't suggest irregular fasting for individuals on the accompanying prescriptions without clinical oversight.

• High portions of insulin

• Certain prescriptions that lower glucose

• Steroid meds

• Meds that lower pulse

• The OMAD diet, as other discontinuous fasting counts calories, may assist with weight reduction. Be that as it may, since it permits just a single feast in a day, it can make addressing supplement needs troublesome and possibly cause unfavorable well-being impacts. It can likewise be trying for individuals who partake in the social parts of food like family eating times and noon with collaborators, adds Amaral.

• Less prohibitive types of irregular fasting with a more prominent eating period taking into consideration more than one feast or dinner timing would be more doable contrasted with the OMAD diet. Talk with your primary care physician prior to beginning any new eating routine. An enrolled dietitian can likewise give you individualized sustenance guidance, adds Dr. Salge Blake.

Chapter 7

Hypothyroidism

What is hypothyroidism?

Hypothyroidism is a condition where there isn't sufficient thyroid chemical in your circulation system and your digestion dials back.

Hypothyroidism happens when your thyroid doesn't make and deliver enough thyroid chemicals into your body. This makes your digestion delayed down, influencing your whole body. Otherwise called underactive thyroid illness, hypothyroidism is genuinely normal.

The point when your thyroid levels are incredibly low is called myxedema. An intense condition, myxedema can cause serious side effects, including:

• A low internal heat level.

• Weakness.

• Cardiovascular breakdown.

- Disarray.

- Trance state.

This serious sort of hypothyroidism is dangerous.

By and large, hypothyroidism is an entirely treatable condition. It very well may be made do with normal prescriptions and follow-up meetings with your medical care supplier.

How takes care of my thyroid responsibilities?

The thyroid organ is a little, butterfly-formed organ situated toward the front of your neck simply under the voice box (larynx). Picture the center of the butterfly's body focused on your neck, with the wings embracing your windpipe (windpipe). The fundamental occupation of the thyroid is to control your digestion. Digestion is the cycle that your body uses to change food to energy your body uses to work. The thyroid makes the chemicals T4 and T3 to control your digestion. These chemicals work all through the body to advise the body's cells how much energy to utilize. They control your internal heat level and pulse.

At the point when your thyroid works accurately, it's continually making chemicals, delivering them, and afterward making new chemicals to supplant what's been utilized. This keeps your digestion working and your body's all's frameworks under control. How much thyroid chemicals in the circulatory system is constrained by the pituitary organ, which is situated in the focal point of the skull beneath the cerebrum. At the point when the pituitary organ faculties either an absence of thyroid chemical or to an extreme, it changes its own chemical (thyroid invigorating chemical, or TSH) and sends it to the thyroid to adjust the sums.

On the off chance that how much thyroid chemicals is excessively high (hyperthyroidism) or excessively low (hypothyroidism), the whole body is affected.

Who is impacted by hypothyroidism?

Hypothyroidism can influence individuals of any age, sex, and identity. It's a typical condition, especially among ladies over age 60. Ladies are by and large bound to foster hypothyroidism after menopause than prior throughout everyday life.

What's the distinction between hypothyroidism and hyperthyroidism?

In hypothyroidism, the thyroid doesn't make sufficient thyroid chemicals.

The contrast between hypothyroidism and hyperthyroidism is the amount. In hypothyroidism, the thyroid makes almost no thyroid chemicals. On the other side, somebody with hyperthyroidism has a thyroid that makes an excess of thyroid chemicals. Hyperthyroidism includes more elevated levels of thyroid chemicals, which makes your digestion accelerate. In the event that you have hypothyroidism, your digestion dials back.

Numerous things are the inverse of these two circumstances. In the event that you have hypothyroidism, you might struggle with managing the virus. Assuming that you have hyperthyroidism, you may not deal with the intensity. They are inverse limits of thyroid capability. In a perfect world, you ought to be in the center. Medicines for both of these circumstances work to get your thyroid capability as near that center ground as could be expected.

Side Effects And Causes

What causes hypothyroidism?

Hypothyroidism can have an essential driver or an optional reason. An essential driver is a condition that straightforwardly influences the thyroid and makes it make low degrees of thyroid chemicals. An optional reason is something that makes the pituitary organ fizzle, and that implies it can't send thyroid invigorating chemical (TSH) to the thyroid to adjust the thyroid chemicals.

Essential drivers of hypothyroidism are substantially more typical. The most widely recognized of these essential drivers is an immune system condition called Hashimoto's infection. Likewise called Hashimoto's thyroiditis or constant lymphocytic thyroiditis, this condition is innate (went down through a family). In Hashimoto's illness, the body's safe framework assaults and harms the thyroid.

This keeps the thyroid from making and delivering sufficient thyroid chemicals.

The other essential drivers of hypothyroidism can include:

• Thyroiditis (irritation of the thyroid).

• Therapy of hyperthyroidism (radiation and careful evacuation of the thyroid).

• Iodine lack (not having sufficient iodine — a mineral your thyroid purposes to make chemicals - in your body).

• Innate circumstances (an ailment went down through your loved ones).

At times, thyroiditis can occur after a pregnancy (post-pregnancy thyroiditis) or a viral disease.

What causes hypothyroidism in pregnancy?

By and large, ladies with hypothyroidism during pregnancy have Hashimoto's infection. This immune system sickness makes the body's resistant framework assault and harms the thyroid. At the point when that occurs, the thyroid can't deliver and deliver sufficiently high degrees of thyroid chemicals, affecting the whole body. Pregnant individuals with hypothyroidism might feel exceptionally drained, struggle with managing cold temperatures, and experience muscle cramps.

Thyroid chemicals mean a lot to fetal turn of events. These chemicals assist with fostering the cerebrum and sensory system. Assuming you have hypothyroidism, dealing with your thyroid levels during pregnancy is significant. On the off chance that the baby doesn't get sufficient thyroid chemicals during advancement, the cerebrum may not grow accurately and there could be issues later. Untreated or deficiently dealt with hypothyroidism during pregnancy might prompt confusion like an unnatural birth cycle or preterm work.

Does conception prevention influence my thyroid?

At the point when you're on conception prevention pills, the estrogen and progesterone within the pills can influence your thyroid-restricting proteins. This builds your levels. On the off chance that you have hypothyroidism, the portion of your drugs should be expanded while you're utilizing contraception pills. When you quit utilizing contraception pills, the measurement should be brought down.

Could hypothyroidism at any point cause erectile brokenness?

At times, there can be an association between untreated hypothyroidism and erectile brokenness. Low testosterone levels are possible when a problem with the pituitary gland is the cause of your hypothyroidism.

 Treating hypothyroidism can frequently assist with erectile brokenness on the off chance that it was straightforwardly brought about by chemical awkwardness.

What are the side effects of hypothyroidism?

The side effects of hypothyroidism generally foster gradually over the long run - in some cases years. They can include:

• Feeling tired (weariness).

- Encountering deadness and shivering in your grasp.

- Having clogging.

- Putting on weight.

- Encountering irritation all through your body (can incorporate muscle shortcomings).

- Having higher than ordinary blood cholesterol levels.

- Feeling discouraged.

- Being not able to endure cold temperatures.

- skin and hair that are dry and coarse.

- Encountering a diminishing sexual interest.

- Having regular and weighty feminine periods.

- Seeing actual changes in front of you (counting hanging eyelids, as well as puffiness in the eyes and face).

- Your voice becomes hoarser and lower.

- Feeling more absent-minded ("cerebrum haze").

Will hypothyroidism make me put on weight?

On the off chance that your hypothyroidism isn't dealt with, you could put on weight. When you are treating the condition, the weight ought to begin to lower. Be that as it may, you will in any case have to watch your calories and exercise to get in shape. Converse with your medical services supplier about weight reduction and ways of fostering an eating regimen that works for you.

Determination And Tests

How is hypothyroidism analyzed?

It can really be challenging to analyze hypothyroidism on the grounds that the side effects can be effectively mistaken for different circumstances. Assuming you have any of the side effects of hypothyroidism, converse with your medical care supplier. The principal method for diagnosing hypothyroidism is a blood test called the thyroid invigorating chemical (TSH) test. Your medical services supplier may likewise arrange blood tests for conditions like Hashimoto's illness. In the event that the thyroid is extended, your supplier might have the option to feel it during an actual test during an arrangement.

The executives And Treatment

How is hypothyroidism treated?

Much of the time, hypothyroidism is treated by supplanting how much chemical your thyroid is making. This is normally finished with a medicine. One medicine that is ordinarily utilized is called levothyroxine. Taken

This medication evens out your levels by increasing the amount of thyroid chemical your body generates orally.

Hypothyroidism is a sensible infection. Notwithstanding, you should consistently accept drugs to standardize how much chemicals are in your body until the end of your life. With cautious administration, and follow-up meetings with your medical services supplier to ensure your therapy is working appropriately, you can have a typical and solid existence.

What occurs on the off chance that hypothyroidism isn't dealt with?

Hypothyroidism can turn into a serious and dangerous ailment in the event that you don't seek treatment from a medical care supplier. On the off chance that you are not treated, your side effects can turn out to be more extreme and can include:

• Creating psychological wellness issues.

• Experiencing difficulty relaxing.

• Not having the option to keep an ordinary internal heat level.

• Having heart issues.

• Fostering a goiter (development of the thyroid organ).

You can likewise foster a serious ailment called myxedema extreme lethargies. When hypothyroidism is not treated, this may occur.

Will I have a similar portion of prescription for hypothyroidism my whole life?

The portion of your drug can really change over the long run. At various places in your day-to-day existence, you might have to have the measures of medicine changed so it deals with your side effects. This could happen in light of things like weight gain or weight reduction. Your levels should be observed all through your life to ensure your drug is working accurately.

Anticipation

Could hypothyroidism at any point be forestalled?

Hypothyroidism can't be forestalled. The most effective way to forestall fostering a serious type of condition or having the side effects influence your life in a serious manner is to look for indications of hypothyroidism. Assuming that you experience any of the side effects of hypothyroidism, the best thing to do is discuss it with your medical care supplier. Hypothyroidism is entirely sensible assuming you get it early and start treatment.

Living With

Are there any food varieties I can eat to help my hypothyroidism?

Most food sources in Western eating regimens contain iodine, so you don't need to stress over your eating regimen. Iodine is a mineral that helps your thyroid produce chemicals. That's what one thought is assuming you have low degrees of thyroid chemical, eating food varieties wealthy in iodine could assist with expanding your chemical levels. The most dependable method for expanding your chemical levels is with a physician-endorsed prescription from your medical services supplier. Attempt no new eating regimens without conversing with your supplier first. It's critical to constantly have a discussion prior to beginning another eating routine, particularly on the off chance that you have an ailment like hypothyroidism.

Food sources that are high in iodine include:

• Eggs.

• Dairy items.

- Meat, poultry, and fish.

- Palatable kelp.

- Iodized salt.

Work with your medical services supplier or a nutritionist (a medical care supplier who has practical experience in food) to create a feast plan. Your food is your fuel. Ensuring you are eating food sources that will help your body, alongside accepting your drugs as educated by your medical care supplier, can keep you solid over the long run. Individuals with thyroid conditions shouldn't consume a lot of iodine in light of the fact that the impact might be dumbfounding (self-disconnected).

Could hypothyroidism at any point disappear all alone?

In a few gentle cases, you might not have side effects of hypothyroidism or the side effects might blur over the long run. In different cases, the side effects of hypothyroidism will disappear soon after you start treatment. For those with especially low degrees of thyroid chemicals, hypothyroidism is a deep-rooted condition that should be dealt with in medicine on a normal timetable.

Chapter 8

Prolon fasting

What is the Fasting Imitating Diet?

The Fasting Copying Diet was made by Dr. Valter Longo, an Italian scientist, and specialist.

He looked to duplicate the advantages of fasting while as yet furnishing the body with sustenance. His changes stay away from the calorie hardship related to different sorts of fasting.

The Fasting Copying Diet or "quick impersonating" is a kind of irregular fasting. Notwithstanding, it varies from additional conventional kinds, like the 16/8 strategy.

The Fasting Impersonating convention depends on many years of examination, including a few clinical investigations.

However anybody can follow the standards of quick mirroring, Dr. Longo sells a five-day get-healthy plan called the ProLon Fasting Copying Diet through L-Nutra, a nourishment innovation organization that he began .

How can it function?

The ProLon Fasting Emulating Diet plan incorporates five-day, prepackaged dinner packs.

All feasts and bites are entirely food determined and plant-based. The dinner units are low in carbs and protein yet high in solid fats like olives and flax.

During the five-day time frame, calorie counters just consume what's held inside the feasting pack.

The very beginning of the eating regimen gives roughly 1,090 kcal (10% protein, 56% fat, 34% carbs), while days two through five give just 725 kcal (9% protein, 44% fat, 47% carbs).

The low-calorie, high-fat, low-carb content of the feast makes your body produce energy from noncarbohydrate sources after glycogen stores are drained. This interaction is called gluconeogenesis.

As per one review, the eating regimen is intended to give 34-54% of typical calorie consumption.

This calorie limitation impersonates the body's physiological reaction to customary fasting strategies, like cell recovery, diminished aggravation, and fat misfortune.

ProLon suggests that all health food nuts counsel a clinical expert — like a specialist or enlisted dietitian — prior to beginning the five-day quick.

The ProLon five-day plan is certainly not a one-time scrub and should be followed each one to a half year to get ideal outcomes.

Synopsis

The ProLon Fasting Emulating Diet is a low-calorie, five-day eating program intended to advance weight reduction and give similar advantages as more conventional fasting strategies.

sources of food to consume and steer clear of

The ProLon dinner pack is separated into five individual boxes — one box each day — and remembers a diagram with proposals for what food sources to eat and the request where to eat them.

A particular mix of food is accommodated breakfast, lunch, supper, and tidbits, contingent upon the day.

The exceptional mix of supplements and decrease in calories is intended to fool your body into believing it's fasting, despite the fact that it's being given energy.

Since calories fluctuate between days, weight watchers actually should don't blend food varieties or convey food sources over into the following day.

All food sources are veggie lovers, as well as gluten and lactose. The bought unit accompanies nourishing realities.

A five-day ProLon Fasting Emulating Diet pack incorporates:

• Nut bars. Feast bars are produced using macadamia nut margarine, honey, flax, almond dinner, and coconut.

• Algal oil. A vegan-based supplement that gives calorie counters 200 mg of the omega-3 unsaturated fat DHA.

• Soup mixes. A blend of enhanced soups including minestrone, minestrone quinoa, mushroom, and tomato soup.

• Home-grown tea. Spearmint, hibiscus, and lemon-spearmint tea.

• Dim chocolate fresh bar. A pastry bar made with cocoa powder, almonds, chocolate chips, and flax.

• Kale wafers. A blend of fixings including flax seeds, healthful yeast, kale, spices, and pumpkin seeds.

• Olives. Olives are incorporated as a high-fat bite. One pack is given on the very first moment, while two packs are given on days two through five.

• NR-1. A powdered vegetable enhancement that conveys a portion of nutrients and minerals that you wouldn't regularly consume during a conventional quick.

• L-Drink. This glycerol-put-together caffeinated drink is given with respect to days two through five when your body has begun gluconeogenesis (starts to make energy from noncarbohydrate sources, like fats).

Weight Watchers are urged to just eat what is held inside the feasting pack and to try not to eat some other food varieties or drinks with two exemptions:

• Soups can be enhanced with new spices and lemon juice.

• Calorie counters are urged to remain hydrated with plain water and decaffeinated teas during the five-day quick.

Outline

The ProLon dinner pack contains soups, olives, homegrown teas, nut bars, nourishing enhancements, chocolate bars, and caffeinated drinks. Health food nuts are urged to just eat these things during their five-day quick.

What are the advantages?

Dissimilar to most of the diets available, the ProLon Fasting Copying Diet is upheld by research.

Additionally, different exploration studies have shown the medical advantages of comparative fasting strategies.

May advance weight reduction

A little report driven by Dr. Longo looked at individuals who finished three patterns of the ProLon Fasting Mirroring Diet north of 90 days to a benchmark group.

Members in the fasting bunch lost a normal of 6 pounds (2.7 kg) and experienced more noteworthy decreases in stomach fat than the benchmark group.

However this study was little and driven by the designer of the ProLon Fasting Emulating Diet, different examinations have shown that fasting techniques are successful in advancing weight reduction.

For instance, one 16-week concentrate on stout men found that the people who rehearsed irregular fasting lost 47% more weight than the individuals who constantly confined calories.

Additionally, extremely low-calorie eats have been demonstrated to support weight reduction.

In any case, proof that the ProLon Fasting Imitating Diet is more powerful than other low-calorie diets or it is at present lacking quick techniques.

May decrease glucose and cholesterol levels

A similar little review driven by Dr. Longo that connected quick copying to fat misfortune likewise saw that the Fasting Imitating Diet bunch encountered a huge drop in glucose and cholesterol levels.

Cholesterol was decreased by 20 mg/dl in those with elevated cholesterol levels, while glucose levels dropped into the ordinary reach in members who had high glucose toward the start of the review.

These outcomes were likewise exhibited in creature studies.

Four days of the eating routine consistently for 60 days provoked recovery of harmed pancreatic cells, advanced solid insulin creation, diminished insulin opposition, and prompted more steady degrees of blood glucose in mice with diabetes.

Albeit these outcomes are promising, more human examinations are expected to decide the eating regimen's effect on glucose.

May diminish aggravation

Studies have shown that discontinuous fasting diminishes markers of irritation, like C-responsive protein (CRP), growth putrefaction factor-alpha (TNF-α), interferon-gamma (ifnγ), leptin, interleukin 1 beta (IL-1β), and interleukin 6 (IL-6).

In a concentrate on individuals rehearsing substitute day fasting for the strict occasion of Ramadan, proinflammatory cytokines were essentially lower during the other day fasting period, contrasted with the prior weeks or later.

One creature investigation discovered that the Fasting Copying Diet might be powerful at decreasing specific incendiary markers.

Mice with different sclerosis were put on either the Fasting Mirroring Diet or a ketogenic diet for 30 days.

The mice in the fasting bunch had essentially lower levels of ifnγ and the T assistant cells Th1 and Th17 proinflammatory cells related to immune system illness.

May slow maturing and cognitive deterioration

One of the primary reasons Dr. Longo fostered the Fasting Copying Diet was to slow the maturing system and chance of specific infections by elevating the body's capacity to self-fix through cell recovery.

Autophagy is a cycle wherein old, harmed cells are reused to create new, better ones.

Irregular fasting has been displayed to enhance autophagy, which might safeguard against cognitive deterioration and slow cell maturing.

A concentrate in mice found that momentary food limitation prompted a sensational increment of autophagy in nerve cells.

One more concentrate in rodents with dementia showed that other day food hardship for a very long time prompted more noteworthy decreases in oxidative harm to mind tissue and diminished mental deficiencies contrasted with a control diet.

Other creature studies have shown that fasting expands the age of nerve cells and improves mind capability.

Furthermore, irregular fasting has been displayed to diminish insulin-like development factor (IGF-1) a chemical that, at undeniable levels, can expand the gamble of specific malignant growth, like bosom disease.

In any case, more human examinations should be completed to completely comprehend what fasting might mean for maturing and sickness risk.

Synopsis

The Fasting Imitating Diet might advance weight reduction, improve autophagy, and diminish glucose, cholesterol, and aggravation.

Who ought to keep away from the fasting impersonating diet?

ProLon doesn't prescribe its eating regimen to specific populations, for example, pregnant or breastfeeding ladies and people who are underweight or malnourished.

Individuals who are adversely affected by nuts, soy, oats, sesame, or celery/celeriac ought to likewise stay away from the ProLon dinner pack as it contains these fixings.

Furthermore, ProLon cautions anybody with ailments like diabetes or kidney sickness to utilize the arrangement under a specialist's management as it were.

Irregular fasting may likewise not be suitable for those with a background marked by disarranged eating.

Outline

Pregnant or breastfeeding ladies and those with sensitivities and certain ailments ought to stay away from this eating regimen.

Would it be advisable for you to attempt it?

The Fasting Copying Diet is doubtlessly ok for sound people and may give a few medical advantages.

Be that as it may, it's muddled whether it's more viable than other, more explored techniques for irregular fastings, like the 16/8 strategy.

The 16/8 strategy is a kind of discontinuous fasting that limits eating to eight hours out of every day, with no nourishment for the excess 16 hours. This cycle can be rehashed more than once each week or consistently, contingent upon individual inclination.

In the event that you have the assets and the self-control to follow the five-day, low-calorie fasting plan from ProLon, it very well might be a decent decision.

That's what simply recollect like other fasting techniques this diet should have proceeded with a long haul to receive the possible rewards.

It's feasible to quickly copy without utilizing the ProLon prepackaged feast pack.

Those with nourishment information can make their own high-fat, low-carb, low-protein, calorie-controlled, five-day feast plan.

Some quick mirroring dinner plans are accessible on the web however they don't convey similar sustenance as the ProLon feast pack which might be the way into the eating regimen's viability.

For those keen on attempting discontinuous fasting, a more explored, practical arrangement, similar to the 16/8 strategy, might be a superior decision.

Outline

For those intrigued by discontinuous fasting, the 16/8 technique might be a more financially savvy decision than ProLon.

The main concern

The ProLon Fasting Emulating Diet is a high-fat, low-calorie discontinuous fasting diet that might advance fat misfortune and decrease glucose, irritation, and cholesterol — like other fasting strategies.

All things considered, just a single human review has been done to date, and more exploration is expected to approve its advantages.

Chapter 9

High fiber foods

What Is Fiber?

Fiber is a kind of toxic supplement that is moved in plant foods.1 Not at all like different supplements, your body can't process or retain fiber, so it goes through your small digestive tract into your digestive organ generally intact.2

Despite the fact that you can't process fiber, this supplement assumes a basic part in well-being. Dietary strands are ordered in view of their dissolvability in water.

There are two fundamental classes of fiber: **dissolvable and insoluble.**

Solvent Fiber

Solvent filaments break up in the water and can be aged or separated by your digestive microbes, which deliver gas as well as advantageous mixtures called short-chain unsaturated fats (SCFAs). Wellsprings of dissolvable fiber incorporate oats, organic products, and beans. There are various classifications of solvent fiber, each with various impacts on health:3

• Solvent, gooey/gel-shaping, promptly aged filaments: These strands thicken in water and are handily matured by stomach microscopic organisms. Models incorporate beta-glucans tracked down in oats.

• Dissolvable, gooey/gel-shaping, non-matured strands: These filaments thicken in water but are impervious to aging. Models incorporate psyllium husk.

• Solvent, nonviscous, promptly aged filaments: These strands disintegrate in the water yet don't thicken. They are effectively matured by stomach microorganisms. Models incorporate inulin and wheat dextrin.

Insoluble Fiber

Insoluble fiber doesn't disintegrate and is inadequately aged by stomach microorganisms. This kind of fiber goes through your stomach-related framework unblemished.

Insoluble fiber is moved in food sources like entire grains, nuts, and seeds.

Most entire food varieties contain a mix of insoluble and dissolvable filaments, yet some are more packed in one than the other. Fiber supplements generally contain one kind of fiber, for example, psyllium husk, which is a sort of solvent fiber.

Why Is Fiber Significant?

Fiber is notable for its positive effect on the stomach-related framework, however, it benefits well-being in alternate ways, as well.

Works on Stomach related Wellbeing

Both insoluble and dissolvable fiber assist you with having agreeable and customary defecations.

Insoluble fiber builds up your crap and advances agreeable solid discharges, while dissolvable fiber draws in water to your stool, which helps keep it delicate and simple to pass.

At the point when the dissolvable fiber is matured by your stomach microorganisms, it produces intensifies called short-chain unsaturated fats (SCFAs, for example, butyrate, acetic acid derivation, and propionate.5 SCFAs emphatically influence stomach well-being in various ways by sustaining digestive cells, managing gastrointestinal irritation, and reinforcing the stomach lining.

Counting calories high in fiber can likewise help forestall and deal with stomach-related conditions like clogging and diverticular disease.

Diminishes the Gamble of Specific Medical issues

Following a high-fiber diet could assist with decreasing your gamble of various medical issues, including colon malignant growth, coronary illness, and type 2 diabetes.1

Fiber is significant for directing gastrointestinal irritation, advancing a sound body weight, and decreasing cholesterol levels, which are all basic for bringing down sickness risk.1 Review discoveries propose that individuals with high fiber admission might have up to a

21% diminished hazard of colon malignant growth contrasted with individuals with low fiber intake.7

In addition, individuals who eat more fiber will generally live longer than individuals who follow low-fiber diets.

Advances a Sound Body Weight

Fiber helps you feel full and fulfilled in the wake of eating, which could assist you with keeping a sound body weight. Solvent fiber dials back your processing and the assimilation of supplements, which assists you with feeling full for longer.

A recent report that included 345 individuals viewed that when, contrasted with any remaining dietary parts, fiber admission was the most grounded indicator of weight reduction. Eats are less connected to sound body weight like the Mediterranean eating routine and plant-based consume fewer calories and are high in fiber-rich food sources like beans, vegetables, natural products, and nuts.

Further develops Cholesterol

Having elevated cholesterol levels has been related to an expanded gamble of coronary illness. Luckily, following a nutritious, high-fiber diet can assist with advancing sound blood lipid levels and safeguard your heart.

Fiber helps decline cholesterol ingestion by the body and expands its discharge. For this reason, following a high-fiber diet has been displayed to bring down blood levels of cholesterol and lessen coronary illness risk.

In a 2017 umbrella survey of 31 meta-examinations, each of the remembered investigations tracked down critical decreases for coronary illness, stroke, and passing from coronary illness while looking at the most elevated versus least dietary fiber intake.

High-Fiber Food Sources and Type 2 Diabetes: What to Be Aware

What Food Sources Are High in Fiber?

There are a lot of fiber-rich food sources that suit practically every dietary preference.

Vegetables

• Crushed yam: 8.2 grams of fiber per cup

• Artichokes: 6.84 grams per medium-sized artichoke

• Brussels sprouts: 6 grams of fiber for each cup

• Collard greens: 6 grams of fiber for each cup

• Broccoli: 5.14 grams of fiber per cup

Natural products

• Avocadoes: 13.5 grams of fiber per avocado

• Raspberries: 9.75 grams of fiber per cup

• Guava: 8.9 grams of fiber per cup

• Blackberries: 7.63 grams per cup

• Pear: 7.13 grams of fiber per cup

Entire Grains

• Teff: 7 grams of fiber for each cup

• Grain: 5.97 grams of fiber per cup

• Quinoa: 5.18 grams of fiber per cup

• Oats: 3.98 grams of fiber per cup

• Earthy colored rice: 3.12 grams of fiber per cup

Nuts and seeds

• Chia seeds: 9.75 grams of fiber per ounce

• Ground flax seeds: 8 grams for each 30-gram serving

• Almonds: 3.5 grams per ounce

• Sunflower seeds: 3.26 grams of fiber per ounce

• Walnuts: 2.72 grams of fiber per ounce

Vegetables

• Naval force beans: 19 grams of fiber for each cup

• Lentils: 15.6 grams per ½ cup

• Dark beans: 15 grams of fiber for each cup

• Kidney beans: 13.1 grams of fiber per cup

• Chickpeas: 12.5 grams of fiber per cup

Other High-fiber Food Varieties

• Cacao nibs: 8 grams of fiber for every ounce

• Psyllium husk powder: 7 grams of fiber for every tablespoon

- Coconut pieces: 6 grams of fiber for each half cup

- 80% dim chocolate: 3.99 grams of fiber per ounce

- Grown grain bread: 2.99 grams of fiber per cut

How Much Fiber Do You Want?

Your fiber needs to rely upon your orientation and age. Here are the ongoing everyday fiber proposals from the US Establishment of Medication (IOM):1

Age Female Male

1-3 years 14 grams 14 grams

4-8 years 16.8 grams 19.6 grams

9-13 years 22.4 grams 25.2 grams

14-18 years 25.2 grams 30.8 grams

19-50 years 25 grams 38 grams

51 and older 21 grams 30 grams

Raising a ruckus around town about everyday fiber consumption for your orientation and age can assist with supporting general well-being and decrease the gamble of ailments like coronary illness, colon malignant growth, and type 2 diabetes.

Sadly, on the grounds that the typical American eating routine is high in super-handled food and low in fiber-rich food varieties like vegetables and organic products, the vast majority don't verge on gathering these proposals. As a matter of fact, the normal American consumes only 15 grams of fiber for every day.

A huge 2022 investigation of 86,642 U.S. grown-ups observed that those with a higher admission of dietary fiber were at an essentially lower hazard of death from all causes, including coronary illness and disease-related passing, contrasted with members with a lower fiber intake. Nonetheless, a 2015 survey of 17 examinations observed that there was a 10% decrease in death from all reasons for every 10-gram per-day expansion in fiber intake.

This implies that regardless of whether your ongoing eating regimen needs fiber, you can without much of a stretch decrease your gamble of various medical issues by getting a charge out of more fiber-rich food varieties. While expanding your fiber consumption, do so sluggishly. Expanding your fiber consumption excessively fast could cause stomach-related side effects like bulging and gas.

A Speedy Survey

Eating more fiber-rich food sources is a brilliant method for advancing stomach-related well-being and lessening your gamble of ailments like coronary illness, clogging, and colon malignant growth.

In the event that your ongoing eating regimen is deficient with regard to fiber, take a stab at picking a couple of the fiber-rich food varieties recorded in this article and gradually adding them to your day-to-day eating design.

Conclusion

The book explains And expatiates better on how the Human growth hormone (HGH), a crucial protein hormone that affects development, metabolism, weight reduction, and muscular strength, rise when fasting. It also let us know the types and benefits of fasting in each phases accordingly.